Goodbye My Friend

Elizabeth Schaufelberger Foley

AuthorHouse™
1663 Liberty Drive, Suite 200
Bloomington, IN 47403
www.authorhouse.com
Phone: 1-800-839-8640

First published by AuthorHouse 11/3/2008

ISBN: 978-1-4389-2651-3 (sc)

*Printed in the United States of America
Bloomington, Indiana*

This book is printed on acid-free paper.

This book is dedicated, with deepest love, to my
children, Kathryn, Stephen and William.

Acknowledgements

This book is the personal journal that I kept during a very difficult time in my life. It began when my husband was admitted to Memorial Sloan-Kettering Cancer Center in New York City for the treatment of Chronic Myelogenous Leukemia (CML) in 1997. He did not know that I recorded our day to day activities, no matter how dull or pointless. I promised myself that when he came home he could read these entries and never feel as if he missed any of the family happenings.

I would like to take this opportunity to thank Memorial Sloan-Kettering Cancer Center and all of the wonderful doctors, nurses and staff that touched my heart and my life. You were all so incredible in your own way. Thank you.

I'd like to express my heartfelt appreciation to my sister, Pat Higgins and to my brother-in-law, Charles Higgins (Butch), who were always there for my children and for me with their exceptional support.

I am grateful to Grace Kelly, a true friend for always being so warm, generous and available.

I began my journal after a conversation with my husband, Willie, before he went into the hospital. He said he was so afraid to miss the day to day happenings of the family. What I found out later was that this silly, meaningless journal kept me going during this time. I found that this was also a calming mechanism for me years later and a way to remember events that were then just a blur.

Introduction

More Than Just A Mother

By: Kathy Schaufelberger

More than just a mother, she is a bedside nurse, a working woman, and a best friend. My mother, Elizabeth Schaufelberger, is one of the strongest people we could ever know.

When we sat down to talk about what was presently happening to this family, she was very confident. A rather conservative lady, she has her head on her shoulders, while she juggles her three children, her sick husband, and herself in her heart.

Her husband (and my father), William Schaufelberger, was diagnosed with leukemia (CML) in 1994. She has been there for her children through it all. From explaining to us what his disease was to having fundraisers for him, she was always there for us. She helps us with homework, friends and family.

She grew up in Morristown, New Jersey and Denville, New Jersey. She met my father in 1974. They married four years later. She works at the Morris County Prosecutor's Office. The people at her office have been really supportive. They have been donating their sick and vacation time to my mother so she can go see Dad.

She goes on to talk about her most trying time, which is right now. My father had a bone marrow transplant in the beginning of October. He was home here, in this germfree sanctuary by November.

It is now the middle of February and he is back at Memorial Sloan-Kettering Cancer Center, because he had a fever.

"He has been there for two weeks now; and they still don't know what's wrong with him," she says with a tear rolling down her cheek.

I just wanted to hug her. She sounded like such a little child. She was confused and hurt, but she knew she had to be strong to keep us strong.

Normally a calm, passive woman, my mother is somewhat rushed through this interview. She smiles, and says that she must pick my youngest brother up from hockey practice, drive my other brother to work, stop at the bank, clean the bathrooms and get to the hospital all before rush hour.

NOTE: This was a Language Arts assignment of Kathryn Schaufelberger during her junior year of high school.

Book 1

October 1, 1997

Dearest Will –

I'm home now – finally sitting after our long first day. It is 11:20 PM and boy do I miss you. I can't seem to stop crying. I hate this. I promised myself that I would write to you each day so that you don't feel left out.

Remember today? It started with radiation – oncology. They set you up with a shield for your lungs. Then we went and saw the dentist. You told me he was some character. While you were with the dentist I received a call from Radiology. They need to make shields for your liver and kidney – so back we went.

After we finished there you didn't want to check in so we went to lunch at Peter's – the little place on the corner. You sure know how to stall when you want to! Finally we did check into Admissions, I guess around 1:15 PM. Pat Walker took us up to your room 1122A. Nice view of York Street, the Park and the 59th Street Bridge.

Now it starts. We must have had 10 different people come in and talk to us today. I know my head is spinning.

You started with Ara-C at 8:00 PM – this is all you get today. Alex came to visit and drove home with me. Really, Alex drove home. I was exhausted.

Butch was here when I got home. Stephen had Matt and Phil over and Will was here too. Kathy was out, but stopped by earlier. I paged her and she was at Rocky's house and will be home soon. I talked to Mom, Pat, Grace and Kristin. I'll write tomorrow.

Good night – Love ya –

Betty

October 2, 1997

Love –

It seems strange to call you that (Love), but that is exactly all I feel for you right now. It is 11:15 PM and I'm just starting to slow down. The dishwasher is almost done and I don't like to go to bed until it is finished.

The kids were off from school today – Rosh Hashanah. I took Stephen to Florham Park this morning, then went up to Morristown with Will to have his glasses adjusted. I then went to the bank, Will's haircut, NJ Pet Supply (Breath Eze for Magic), Sports Authority and Foodtown. I came home and straightened things out – saw Kathy for a bit and left to come see you. I made it to the hospital in about 1 hour 15 minutes. Things are starting to happed to you. You woke up this morning feeling fine but by the time I arrived both your head and stomach were bothering you. Your head was really hurting. Julie (nurse) came in and gave you something but you got sick shortly after receiving it. Julie gave you more. I bought some things from home today. Lamp, clock radio and pictures, your room is starting to look better.

The 2:00 PM chemo seems to make you very tired – you try to fight it because I am there. Sleep, your body is telling you something. I left somewhat early. I guess about 6:45 PM (I'm afraid to walk in the dark). I was home by 8:00 PM.

Stephen and I ran out for your birthday gifts. Will is

over Dan S. house because Kristen is there. I'm picking him up at 9:00 PM. Kathy is at work and will be home by 10:15 PM. I tried calling you a number of times, but you're not answering. Stephen has been trying to reach you and is getting upset. He thinks something is wrong. I told him that either you turned off the phone, are sleeping or in the bathroom. I called again a little after 10:00 PM — but received a recording that all phones are shut off for patient comfort. I guess that is a good idea.

Talked to Sandy, Kristin, Anne, Pat, Al and Joanne, and Edie. Alex called your room while I was there.

See you soon Love,

Betty

October 3, 1997

Willie —

Happy 50th Birthday!!!   I'm sorry — it won't be so
happy. I called you early this morning, before Kathy and
Stephen left for school. You already sounded terrible.
The kids went to school for half a day and I bought
them in to see you. You slept a lot, but you need that.
Every time you sat up you would get sick. I feel so bad
and helpless. We bought you balloons, CD walkman and
some CDs. You're not really interested right now.

I took the kids upstairs to the Rec. Room. Stephen
and Will played a few games of pool. Kathy and I just
sat and watched. This seems to be hitting Kathy the
hardest. She hates to see you sick.

We were going to have cake with you at 3:30 PM
— Julie was going to bring it in. The nurses got an ice
cream cake from downstairs. You were so sick that you
asked me to leave by 3:15 PM. Maybe we'll have cake
tomorrow. We made it home by 4:45 PM.

Lana came over and I drove in with her to see you.
We picked up Alex and came to visit for about a half
hour. They have you on morphine for the headache but
it doesn't seem to be helping. No one seems to know
where the headaches are coming from. Lana and Alex
bought you a few gag gifts. Alex drove home. I was
just too tired. The kids were all out at different
places. I decided to get the floor washed tonight. One

less thing to do tomorrow. Stephen put the wash away for me – it really is a help.

Calls tonight were from Teresa, Sandy, Avi, Ted, Helen N., Diane, Pat and Grace.

I'm falling asleep here, so I'm signing off now and will talk to you again soon.

Love,

Betty

October 5, 1997 for Oct 4, 1997

Will -

I never sat down last night to write - so I'm writing first thing Sunday morning. I was supposed to get Stephen up for work at about 7:15 AM. My alarm went off and I guess I turned it off. I woke up at 7:52 AM - We made it to work by 8:00 AM.

Anyway, yesterday was another long day - I started to clean the house (something that I can't seem to put my mind to right now), went to Foodtown (Scott R. was asking about you), came home and Pat was here. Grace came a little later and we left to come see you. Grace drove.

When we first got there you really weren't feeling too good. You still haven't eaten - Friday and now Saturday. You still have a fever, nauseous and vomiting. We sat with you for about an hour or so and then went for a walk and had some lunch. I had Nachos Grande. Then we came back.

You looked better when we got back. You said you had just gotten sick again, but you're not as flushed and you seem to be more awake. You seemed anxious to shower, so we left about a half hour later.

I called you around 9:00 PM and you sounded like my old Willie. You sounded as you would sound answering the phone at home. We talked a bit and you hung up.

The kids, (Stephen and Will) were skateboarding in the driveway when we came home with some friends. Kathy is over at Joe's house. Will slept over at Dan S. house and both Kathy and Stephen were home early tonight (11:00 PM and 11:30 PM). Even though I'm exhausted for some reason I decided to clean our room and change things around. I finally went to bed at 12:30 AM. I better get myself into a routine and slow down before I get sick myself. Well, I better get this day started and I'll see you later.

Lots of Love

Betty

October 5, 1997

Willie –

I fell asleep and never wrote anything last night – Today
is Oct 6, 1997.

October 6, 1997

My Dear Will –

Right now it is 11:00 PM and I want to make sure I write before I fall asleep.

I came in to see you today around noon and I left about 4:30 PM. Today started radiation. You had a tough time this morning. You vomited six times during your first treatment. This afternoon you had no problem.

Kenny stopped by for a short visit. Wanted to know if you were going to Florida in March to play golf.

I got home by 6:00 PM or so. Butch was here and cooked dinner. Both Kathy and Stephen worked today. It seems like I had a million calls today. Joanne, Pat, Grace, Kristin, Nancy and Joe, Diane, Barbara W, my Mom, your Mom. I called Ted, Lana and Rose.

When I talked to Joe S. he asked me questions and said that by this time his brother had already started to deteriorate. I truly feel you will come through this like a champ. We'll just take one day at a time.

I love you,
Betty

October 7, 1997

My Love –

I just finished talking to you. Stephen and Will talked to you too. Kathy is still at work. I really miss you (I'm crying again). I didn't get to see you for too long today. I came in around 11:15 AM but had to leave by 1:30 PM. Will had an orthodontist appointment. I wasn't too much fun today. I came in, talked a few minutes and took a nap on the extra bed in your room. I'm so tired. Today started isolation. I guess you'll get used to me with a mask on. I hate the gloves. Your hands sweat so much. The ride home was quick. I was home before Will was home from school.

I grabbed dinner with Kristin tonight. We went to Holihans, nothing exciting, but it was good to see her.

Mike, my brother called to see how you were doing. Diane called (while I was out), your mother called (wants me to bring her in on Thursday), Maggie, Lana, Teresa and Maria also called.

I'm going to have my coffee and watch a little tv. (I don't like doing that without you either).

I love you –

Betty

October 8, 1997

My Sweet Will –

For some reason today was tougher than most. I really don't know why. You seemed more emotional today than usual. You told me how when you go down for your radiation treatments you listen to Kenny G. and think about the two of us in a field of flowers. It will happen – we'll find that field. I promise. I also saw you crying twice today, but I didn't say anything, mainly because I knew I would start crying too.

Ted came and gave platelets today and then came up to visit for a little bit. He stayed until 3:00 PM. I only stayed until a little after 4:00 PM. They came and took you for your last radiation treatment. I hate leaving you. It hurts.

I got a lot of calls today, Teresa, Pat, my Mom, Mary Diane, Joe, Gleek, Bill (he called you too), Anne, JBD and Grace.

Well – I think I need some sleep – so bye for now – I love you,

Betty

October 9, 1997

Willie –

It's pretty late so this letter might end up short. Today Pat drove in to give platelets for you. We both came up to visit first for an hour or so then at about 1:15 PM I took Pat to the Donor Room. I then came back to you and for some reason all of a sudden you were sick.

Pat came back around 4:30 PM, visited a little bit and we left. Kathy worked today (Pat and I went to watch her work); Stephen went to open gym and Will was home. After Stephen came home he needed help typing a chemistry lab and then some computer management stuff.

Received calls from Anne, Mary, Terri, Kristin, Lana and Debbie.

We're still trying to figure out when the transplant is. I really would like to be there. From what you are telling me, it's going to be real early in the morning like 5:00 AM or so. I hope someone can give a more definite time soon.

Good night my Love,

Betty

October 10, 1997

TRANSPLANT DAY

Will –

Good Morning!! I called you about 7:30 AM and you said the doctor was there giving you the new bone marrow. You said there are four tubes. Most people get one to two tubes, but the more you receive the better base for you.

I feel so bad that I'm not there. Had I known it would be 7:00–7:30 AM I could have been there, but since we last thought it would be 5:00 AM I didn't even attempt to come in. I'm sorry.

Well it is now late evening on the 10th. I came in today around 11:15 AM and stayed until 5:00 PM. Traffic was horrible. Al called while I was there and so did Alex, Lana and the kids to see how you did. You asked me today if the kids even miss you. Of course they do!! It's strange not having you here. All three went out tonight so I was home alone – weird. I paid bills, what fun!! I talked to my mother (she sent me a book today), I talked to Grace, Joe S. and Carol C. Everyone wanted to know how you did. I'm going to get some sleep now so – good night.

Love, Betty

October 11, 1997

Will –

I ran around this morning doing regular things like take Kathy to work, NJ Pet Supply, bank and Foodtown. I got the boys situated and left for the hospital with Grace around 11:15 AM.

You seemed to be feeling pretty good. You looked good too. We played cards for a couple of hours and you beat both of us in two games of Rummy 500.

Grace and I left the hospital around 4:30 PM. We went to Jim Johnson's for dinner with Pat and John. I talked to you around 10:00 PM. You seemed extra tired.

You also received blood and platelet transfusions today – you don't like that.

Talk to you tomorrow.

I love you,

Betty

October 12, 1997

Will:

I woke up early today — I wish I could sleep a little. I washed the floors and called you before 8:00 AM. I then did some laundry and started to get ready to come see you. I dropped Will, Joe and Daren off at hockey (18-2). Daren's mom will bring them home. I then came to the hospital. Don and Sandy came by before I got there; but Avi and Debbie stopped by. They stayed about an hour or a little more.

You seem down today. You said you are bored. You can't let this situation get to you — Yeah, it stinks, but it will all be worth it in the end — you'll see.

It's so hard to come see you and not be able to kiss or hug you. (I'm crying again — I'm so weak — I'm such a wimp)!

Pat called today, Kieran took Kathy out driving. Stephanie P, Lana and your Mom called today.

Well, I need to get some rest.

Lots of Love,

Betty

October 13, 1997

Willie:

Happy Columbus Day! Talked to you early this morning and you sounded pretty good. You seemed to be looking forward to the kids coming in. We got in at about 1:20. You didn't touch your lunch — you said your stomach was bothering you.

Stephen started complaining that his stomach hurt while we were walking to the hospital. I think he's nervous. He's so afraid of you getting a germ. Stephen and Will went to the 15th floor to play pool.

You didn't really talk to the kids — if anything you made them uncomfortable. We understand that you are getting depressed — you hate being locked up — you said you feel like you are in jail. We all hate the whole situation, but we also know we have to get through this.

We only stayed for about an hour and a half. The kids didn't say a word — everyone was lost in their own thoughts. You're making things so difficult for all of us.

Mary called early this morning. I also spoke to Lana, Grace, Pat, Maria, Debbie, Joanne B. and Alex. Obviously you have so much to live for, fight for and so much support.

Please open your eyes!

Betty

October 14, 1997

Sweetheart –

I talked to you early. You seem to be a lot better than yesterday. Stephen is home today – he was up and down all night until about 3:30 AM. Boy am I exhausted. I tried to take a nap since I was coming in late today because Alex is coming after work to give blood and I'll drive him home.

I got to the hospital a little before 2:00 PM. You were watching home movies and we did that until about 5:00 PM. Merry has been in and out and then your dinner came. Dr. Young stopped by for a few minutes. After you ate you spent most of your time in the bathroom. Your hair is really falling out now. It will grow back – don't worry. You received a call from three (3) drunk realtors, as you put it. I don't know who they were (I think you said Laurie, Maria and I can't remember the third one).

Alex came up about 7:45 PM. He didn't come in, he was afraid to give you germs. He hopes you understand. I got home at 9:10 PM and kept on going. Stephen wanted clean sheets because he thought germs were on his bed. He needed his raccoon washed and a shirt ironed for school.

Calls today were Lana, Diane, Teresa, Helen N., Karen T., Kieran, Kenny and Mom.

Love you – Betty

October 15, 1997

Love –

Hi! Stephen is home again today. He did get up, shower and eat breakfast, but for some reason he is dizzy and light-headed. I decided to let him stay home for another day. I'll see how he feels later – hopefully better.

Pat came down this morning to come give platelets again. Pat drove into the city. She's getting good. After she gave the platelets she came up to visit for an hour or so.

Kenny came to see you this afternoon so Pat and I left. Traffic was crazy – it took us over two hours to get home.

Stephen still is light-headed and dizzy. I gave him a Benedryl for his hives, but I don't know what to give him for the dizziness. If things aren't better tomorrow, I'll have to bring him to the doctor.

I talked to you around 10:00 PM. You sound real good. Callers for today were Kieran, Lana, Mom, Irene, Bill and Diane.

Good Night –

B

October 16, 1997

Hi Hon –

Today seemed to last forever. Stephen still doesn't
feel good – seems to be mainly light-headed. I made an
appt with Dr. Gonzalez. She feels it is nerves, stress
and maybe a slight inner ear infection that might be
making him dizzy/light-headed. She didn't give him any
antibiotics, just said to take an antihistamine.

I came to see you by 1:00 PM. I stopped by the
Blood Donor Room to say hello to Grace, Ed and Chris.
Only Grace was able to give platelets, the other two had
counts that were too low.

We watched Legal Eagles – good movie.

Cindy came in and talked to us for a while. She
answered a lot of questions. I left around 4:30 PM.
I didn't want to leave. I got home around 6:00 PM.
Butch was still here. We talked until 6:30 and then
he left. I took Stephen to Burlington Coat Factory and
then to Sports Authority. We then came home and I
started helping him with the typing of chemistry stuff. I
finished the wash, did some ironing and talked to Lana,
Anne, Carol C., Grace, Kristin and Pat. You called around
9:30 PM and talked to Stephen and Will. Kathy called
you this afternoon, she's at work until 10:00 PM. I'm
really tired, bye for tonight – I'll write again tomorrow.

Love, B

October 17, 1997

Willie –

I just talked to you. I went to dinner with Grace and Kristin at the "Office". I tried calling you from Grace's at 9:55 PM and the phones were off. I'm really glad you called me. Kathy went to dinner and on the hayride for Merry's birthday. She didn't think it was worth $10.00. She takes her PSAT's tomorrow. She is nervous. Stephen went to the movies and Will stayed home.

I really enjoyed being with you today. Your spirits are good. I miss you here. I really don't like being alone. Hurry home, please.

I'm signing off now because I have to get up early to get Kathy to school.

Lots of Love,

Betty

October 18, 1997

Willie –

It's really October 19, 1997 because it's 12:03 AM and I'm just sitting down. I don't seem to be able to catch up – I am constantly doing something for someone. You really looked good today. Your spirits are good, your head was starting to peel and you kept picking at it. Finally I asked you what you were doing and you said untangling your hair, you felt a knot.

We played cards again and boy did you whip me. I think you won by about 500 points.

I'm cutting this short because I'm beat.

I love you,

Betty

October 19, 1997

Will —

Right now it is 9:45 PM and boy am I <u>still</u> tired. In fact, when I'm done writing I'm going to bed. Will had hockey practice this morning; Stephen worked from 1:00 – 6:00 and Kathy is going out to breakfast and taking it easy — she's tired too.

Pat and Grace came in with me today to visit. Pat and I bought you a puzzle and checkers. You didn't seem too excited. I hate seeing you bored — it really makes you crazy sitting in your room. I wish you would talk to me about visitors. You don't seem as happy when people are here. I wish you could enjoy them because it is support for me.

You called tonight around 9:00 PM and talked to all three kids. They really are concerned — they always ask me how you are as soon as I get home. I heard Stephen ask you how you were doing and he always want to know "did it work?" Will asked you how you are feeling.

I miss you so much here at home. Come Home!!!

Love,

Betty

October 20, 1997

Willie:

What a day this has been. It was really nice at the beginning. I was able to get to you before noon. We worked on the puzzle most of the time, when all of a sudden I realized it was 4:40 PM. I was at the FDR by 5:00 PM or so. When I realized hardly anyone else was on the highway, I turned on the radio and heard that Route 80 was closed both ways. Something to do with hazardous materials mixing together and blowing up. I ended up taking the Parkway South to Route 280 West so it took me about 2½ hours total to get home.

Boy am I beat.

Love you lots,

Betty

October 21, 1997

Will –

Today has already been busy. I cleaned the house, did some laundry, went to the bank, Foodtown, Post Office and work. I also dropped off your absentee ballot. I made it home by 11:00 AM to meet Pat. Pat is giving platelets again. Pat and Butch have been great. We worked on the puzzle for a while, then you felt like beating me in checkers. When Pat came up we played a little cards. Pat won. Our trip home was uneventful. Pat and Butch stayed for dinner. I took Stephen to the mall after open gym. Talked to you around 10:00 PM. I miss you here – I really do!!

Love always,

B–

October 22, 1997

Hon –

I'm writing late tonight. It's 11:25 PM and I'm tired. I sat in traffic coming in this morning. There was a bus fire on Route 80 so the express lanes were closed. Grace called me to tell me not to take Route 80 – I took Route 280 East to the Parkway North. I only sat for 10 minutes or so.

You really look good today. I can't believe how well things are going. I hope they continue. Your white blood count was 300 today! We're on our way up!

Tonight was a "Stephen Fight Night". I need a rest. I feel like I'm being beat up, but I guess I'll get through this. I don't have any choice. A group of people from work came in to give platelets; Darryl N.; Paul S; Bob W and Rich H.

Good night,

Betty

October 23, 1997

Hi Love –

It's almost 11:00 PM, so this will be short, I need some sleep. I can't believe Route 80 today – a tractor trailer (wide load) got wedged underneath a bridge in Wayne and the materials he was carrying fell off so the center and right lanes were closed. Every day is a new experience on "80".

When I came down the FDR they had my exit closed (Exit 13). I don't like looking for new routes.

We finished the puzzle today. You still look great and seem to feel okay too. Maryanne H.; Greg A. and Al M. gave platelets today. Paul M. drove them in, but couldn't give – afraid of needles.

Your count was 600 today. Your hemoglobin and platelets were low, you are getting two transfusions today.

I'm tired – love ya,

Betty

October 24, 1997

Sweetheart:

It's late (12:19 AM) but today, for some reason I'm not tired. I really should be because I was up at 6:30 AM, got the kids out, had coffee, took my shower, talked to you, went to my bank, Foodtown, SoundWaves (had Kathy's CD player installed in her car); went to our bank (PNC); then to Seven-11 (Saw Nancy G. there — she said to say hi) stopped home to drop everything off; took the truck, went to Office Max to have Kathy's second book copied; and then came to see you.

Traffic was actually good — first time this week!

You didn't seem as üp as you have been lately. You seem scared about coming home. It is still some time away. We'll be okay. We'll all be real careful and use a lot of common sense. I can understand your apprehension. Right now you are in a completely secure surrounding. If something goes wrong — you push a button. At home it is up to us.

We played Rummy-O. I won. I got home about 6:10 PM and took Will to a school dance. Stephen went to the homecoming football game and Kathy did her usual, got together with about 6 kids and watched a movie.

I ran out to pick up Kathy's book — what a disaster. I also went to pick up some greeting cards. I came home at around 9:00 PM and then started cleaning (I had sausage and peppers around 10:30 PM). I cleaned the downstairs and the porch. I'll finish the rest tomorrow morning before I come in.

I miss you so much!!!

Love, B

October 25, 1997

Willie —

Today your count was 1.8. You must be feeling better because you yelled at me for moaning on the phone. I guess I was looking for a little compassion and thought maybe I would get it from you. Instead you just asked me why it was taking me so long to clean the house and porch (I want it extra clean for you). Get some sleep and don't try to do too much. I won't complain anymore — I promise. I left here about 12:15 PM and made it to the hospital by 1:30 PM — not bad timing. We watched a family tape and played Rummy-O again. I won. We then played cards — you won! I left about 4:45 PM. I went to Kieran and Barbs for their Halloween party — I wish you were with me. It really is strange to be alone. Pat and Butch went too.

Stephen is out with Wendy. Kathy is out with Merry, Regina, Tom and Rocky. They were going to Chilies' and then to watch a movie at someone's house.

Will was going to sleep over at Dan S. house, but ended up staying home.

You called around 11:30 PM or so. Just checking in. I'll be in by 1:00 PM tomorrow. Pat is giving platelets again.

Love you,

Betty

October 26, 1997

Willie:

Today your count was 2,700. I can't believe it went up almost 1,000 points from yesterday. Your hemoglobin was down and you had another blood transfusion. You said you were getting used to seeing the red stuff hanging.

Pat came in and gave platelets again. Today is Pat's birthday, so I made a cake and we had it with you. You said you really can't taste the chocolate. We watched "Scream" the movie, it was okay.

Nothing else is happening, so I guess I'll sign off.

I love you and wish you were here with me —

Betty

October 27, 1997/October 28, 1997

Love –

Today is really October 28, 1997. I was too tired last night to write.

Driving in today took a little over 2 hours. The George Washington Bridge was backed up between Teaneck and Englewood because of an accident on the Cross Bronx Expressway. What amazed me was after you got through the toll – it was clear sailing.

You seemed very quiet today. I was planning on going to the Family Support Group, but we were watching "Braveheart". We didn't finish watching it because Kenny stopped by and so did Dick J. I left by 4:15 PM and got home by 5:30 PM – good timing. Hardly any traffic.

Kathy worked today and Stephen and Will were here playing basketball. Butch made stew and we ate dinner by 6:00 PM.

I didn't sleep real well last night – I think I woke up almost every hour. I miss having you here.

Love, Betty

October 28, 1997

Hi Hon –

Today was hectic for some reason. I had my hair cut early but noticed the "Check Oil Level" light on the truck. I was going to return Stephen's skis to Pelican today but came home instead and called you about the oil light. You said to go back to Jiffy Lube. They said there are no leaks, but it is down ½ quart. Not to worry about it.

I arrived at the hospital around noon. Your counts were 7,900. Great!!! They took you off your antibiotic and the GFSC (fertilizer stuff). We'll see what your counts are tomorrow.

I got home about 5:40 PM, ate a little dinner, went to Blockbuster to return our movies, Staples with Stephen and Tops to get wires for Play Station. I then went to Grace's for some soup. It was good talking to her. She is so upset with the phones at work and Patty C. I got home before 10:00 PM and called you.

Kathy quit her job. She upsets me so much. She can't seem to handle authority. She wants to work at Jersey Boy. She dropped off her application today. I understand she doesn't like working until 10:00 PM, but come on – she got mad because they changed her schedule – 10:00 AM to 6:00 PM on Saturday. That's when she quit.

Well, I'm going to bed now and hopefully can sleep through the night –

I need you!

Lots of Love,

Betty

October 29, 1997

Willie:

Today had to be the worst yet. As soon as I told you about Kathy quitting her job you got mad. Our visit together was terrible. I hardly talked for fear of saying the wrong thing. You didn't want her to go for her license, etc. Later you called and changed your mind.

Your counts went down today, about half of yesterday. They expected that. They gave you one dose of the GSFC and will see what happens tomorrow.

Our talk this evening was bad too. I guess I'm not handling things too well. You told me I should go see someone or get some medicine to cope.

Hope tomorrow is better.

Betty

October 30, 1997

Will:

I took Kathy to Dr. Connolly today. He feels the thing on Kathy's shoulder and face should come off. We'll see.

I got to you about 2:00 PM today. Things seem better between us. I'm trying my hardest to cope with everything.

Pat called and said she will take one day off next week and help me clean the whole house before you come home. That will be a big help.

Today Ann came in to start talking about how things should be for you when you come home. At times it seems overwhelming, but we'll do it. I'm excited just thinking of you here again.

Love, Betty

October 31, 1997

Hi Hon!

Happy Halloween! I went to Dr. Deane's today. He cleaned me out and gave me a Z-Pak prescription. I talked to him about the stress and coping. He said I can do it — we'll make it.

I came in before noon and we talked and played some cards and Ann came in again to talk. I left about 4:15 PM and didn't get home until after 6:30 PM. Friday traffic stinks! I went out to Jim Johnson's with Grace and came home and cleaned. You called around 11:30 PM. I am extra tired.

I'll see you tomorrow.

Love,

Betty

November 1, 1997

Sweetheart —

Today was real ugly out. It rained all day. It was very windy too. Grace and Pat came to give platelets today but for some reason Pat's iron level was too low. She was mad about that. We visited until 4:20 PM or so and we made it home before 6:00 PM I ordered Chinese food. Grace stayed and Stephen had Matt here.

I went and checked prices on vacuum cleaners. I think I did okay on the one I bought. You called me tonight around 11:15 PM. Tomorrow is the NY Marathon on 1st Avenue and President Bill Clinton is going to be on the west side. "Grid Lock Alert Day". I'm not sure if I'll come in or not. I'm going to the Melissa Neier Foundation Fundraiser at noon. I'll talk to you tomorrow about visitation. I think I'll feel strange if I miss a day.

Love ya,

Betty

November 2, 1997

Willie:

Today was the first day I missed coming in to see you. I didn't like it. I took Will to a hockey game at 9:30 AM and at 11:30 AM I left to go to a Celebrity Brunch for the Melissa Neier's Memorial Fund.

I left there about 2:30 and went to Sears to buy a new Christmas Tree. Then I went home, changed and went to Costco. After I cleaned everything up and put everything away I made dinner. I then started helping Stephen with some typing and did the laundry. I didn't think this day was ever going to end.

I talked to you and all the kids were home early which I'm glad about because now I can go to sleep.

Love ya,

Betty

November 3, 1997

Hon –

Today is Kathy's 17th Birthday and she passed her driving test too! She was so nervous it was almost funny.

I came in to see you around 1:00 PM. We played battleship. Ann came in to talk to us and will again tomorrow. Right now it looks like you might be home by Friday. I hope so.

I'm extra tired so I'm going to sleep now. It's 10:50 pm.

Love,

Betty

November 4, 1997

Will –

Right now it is 11:00 PM and I'm watching the news. Right now the governor's race is 47% McGreevy and 46% – Whitman – this is really nerve-wracking.

Today Ann, RN came in and finished up talking about when you come home. Right now it looks like Friday, November 7, 1997. I am so excited and I hope you are too. We'll take good care of you – I'm tired.

Good night Love,

Betty

November 5, 1997

Will –

Today is the other day I won't be visiting you. Pat and I are going to clean this house real good to make sure there are no germs.

Pat got here before 9:00 AM and started right away. We started in our bedroom and worked our way down. Pat worked me too hard and boy do I ache!!! My hands are worthless.

I asked how you made out today and you said lonely. I'm sorry, but you'll be home soon and you surely won't be lonely here.

I can't believe only "2 more sleeps"!

Love,

Betty

November 6, 1997

Willie —

This should be my last note — you should be here next to me tomorrow. You did it!!! You got through the toughest part, the chemo, the radiation, the transplant and all of the side effects. Now we just have to watch out for germs — bacteria, etc.

I'm so excited —

Love you forever,

Betty

Book 2

Upon his discharge from Memorial Sloan-Kettering Cancer Center Willie had the opportunity to read Book 1 of my journal and enjoyed the entries and could remember the days as he read through the journal.

He never had the opportunity to read Book 2.

Feb 7, 1998 – Feb 11, 1998

Letters in home computer. Computer crashed and I lost all of the letters. (Glad I only lost a few letters – I guess from now on I'll handwrite).

Feb 12, 1998

Will:

It's about 10:30 PM and I can't wait to go to bed (wish you were in it). I'm trying to remember what I did today so I can tell you. This morning I did laundry, went to the post office, my bank, PNC bank, Foodtown and then over to Drug Fair. Oh, I also stopped at Gina's to bring her pot back from the other day when she gave us the soup.

When I got home Grace had just pulled in and we came to visit you. We were at the hospital by about 12:00. When we got there you had just finished your shower. You were really wiped out from that for some reason. You still have your fever and no answers. I'm getting frustrated and can imagine how you feel. I just want to know what's going on. Maybe tomorrow they will have the results from the catheter culture. When your lunch came Grace and I went down to the cafeteria and had a cheeseburger and fries. I felt bad leaving you sitting in your room alone to eat lunch. You already eat breakfast and dinner alone. I don't think I'll ever do that again.

You received a pentamidine (or something like that) treatment today. Grace and I left at about 3:50 PM. Traffic was okay, uneventful.

This evenings calls were Pat, Kristin, Anne, Debbie (Avi's). I called Joanne and Al to let them know where things stand.

You called around 10:10 PM and talked to the kids first. You made a comment that you were going to get answers tomorrow. I hope you do. I'll talk to you in the morning.

Love,

B

Feb 14, 1998/Feb. 16, 1998

Hi! Today is Monday, February 16th. I'm writing whatever I can remember from Saturday. The computer is down and I haven't been writing. Sorry.

Saturday was Valentine's Day. I bought you a card, a balloon and a puzzle you haven't' touched. I've been trying to do it, but I can't help but cheat. (They give you a cheat sheet).

You didn't feel great today, but you couldn't put your finger on exactly what was bothering you. You never got out of bet, but you were awake and talking.

I left here around 4:00 PM. Will had a game this morning and didn't do anything at night. Stephen and Kathy went to Joe's. I went to Grace's for dinner. Pat and Butch and Bonnie and Judy D. were also there for dinner. You told me you would call me at Grace's so I stayed there. You didn't call until 10:45 PM or even a little later. You were really sick at this point (vomiting, diarrhea, temperature of 39.7). I talked to you for about 20 seconds and then you hung up. I called the nurses station to see what was happening and they said it was from the new medication and also they would be giving you a blood transfusion. I left Grace's and was home by 11:15 PM. I couldn't get to sleep until after 2:00 AM. Get better. Hon.

Love you –

Betty

Sunday Feb. 15, 1998

Will —

I spoke to you around 8:00 AM. You really don't sound good. You have chills and a fever of 39.5. I just want to be there with you. I called Pat because I'm worried and scared. She said not to leave yet, she would be down to drive me in. We got to the hospital by 11:15 AM. Pat sat down the hall knitting and reading. I came to visit you. You really don't look too good. You are very flushed and uncomfortable from the fever. I cleaned around your room a little, sat and talked to you a little bit. Around 1:00 PM I went to meet Pat and have a cup of coffee and hopefully let you get some sleep. When I came back you were starting to look a little better. Around 3:00 PM you said to have Pat come in. You definitely have perked up since I got here this morning. Dr. O'Reilly stopped by to see how you are doing. He said the new medicines you are getting for fungus is called the great shake and bake medicine. Shake for chills — Bake for fever. The way I understand it is you will be on this for 7 —10 days.

Another doctor came in and introduced herself as one of the doctors doing the bronchoscopy tomorrow. She explained exactly what they will do. You would not allow them to do a lung biopsy though. I just hope they wont' have to do a lung biopsy three days from now. I hate you to go through this again.

Pat and I left around 4:00 PM. I was home by 5:00 PM and didn't go out again. I did laundry, vacuuming and straightening up. After Kathy and Stephen came home I went right to bed. Talk to you tomorrow.

Love,

B —

February 16, 1998

Will:

Today is Monday - President's Day. The kids don't have school until Wednesday. Kathy is working today. Stephen works tomorrow. I spoke to Dave Beck this morning about the computer. Hopefully it is fixable. He is supposed to stop by sometime between 12 and 1:00 today.

Pat, John and Grace came into the city today. John drove. They wanted to save me the drive and thought I could use some company especially since you were having surgery.

I got to the hospital around noon, you weren't feeling too great. You had the bronchoscopy this morning and they gave you morphine and codeine. You seem pretty much out of it and very tired.

When your lunch came you surprised me and tried to eat a little. You had some soup and a little soda. You said your appetite isn't what it used to be. Will called. He is looking for Dave Beck. He's not too anxious, is he? Dave didn't get to the house until 3:30 PM. He took the computer with him and bought it back at 8:00 PM. It is fine now.

Will was at the mall with Dan when I came home and Kathy and Stephen were at Joe's. I went to Jim Johnson's with John, Pat and Grace.

I talked to you around 10:15 PM. You don't sound too good, but I understand the meds are making your fever rise.

Talk to you in the AM

Love,

B –

February 17, 1998

Willie –

Hi – the kids are still home today. They don't have any specific plans. Kathy is going to go into work early so she can get out earlier. Stephen played basketball with Matt, Rocky and Joe. Will, I guess, will sit at the computer to catch up on his previous withdrawal while it was down.

Pat is stopping at our house around 3:30 PM to make a roast beef. Pat and Butch are always there for me. They're there for you too! Whatever you need. I got home around 5:15 PM or so and I was exhausted – I took a ½ hour nap on the sofa in the family room before dinner. Stress is getting to me. I don't know what's happening to you. No one seems to have any answers. I guess it's frustrating for them too. Julie was talking about some type of a scan they are going to do to you (Lung Gallium Scan). It's with a nuclear die and then they scan you for 3 days and hopefully this will direct them to your infection or whatever.

You were supposed to call me tonight but you felt really lousy and never called. I worried about you all night. I wanted to call the nurses station, but I didn't want to bother them. I'll talk to you tomorrow.

Love Always,

B

February 18, 1998

It's Thursday evening and I forgot to write yesterday, sorry. The days are running into each other so I'll only tell you what I remember.

The kids went back to school. You had a bad day, diarrhea and chills. You didn't eat anything while I was there.

C'mon Hon – FIGHT!!!!!

B

February 19, 1998

Will —

I won't be in until later than normal — Kathy goes to Dr. Connolly today for a biopsy on her shoulder. She was really better than I ever thought she would be. He gave her two needles and she didn't jump or anything. He will have results Tuesday or Wednesday and she gets her stitches removed on Thursday.

I came home from that and went food shopping and then came in to see you. Another tough day for you. You seemed to have horrible chills. You couldn't get rid of them. We did try to play cards — that lasted for 3 hands and you were exhausted. We both took naps. It felt good, except the chair in you room is very uncomfortable. Your mother called while I was there. I left around 5:00 PM since I came in late. Butch stopped by and made Grandma's Chicken for the boys. I had some of that and ran over to Grace's to pick up my paycheck. I wrote a bad check at Foodtown today and I want to get some money in that account.

I called you tonight — your spirits are going downhill — you better start fighting or change your attitude!!!! You moaned most of this evening's conversation. Let's go.

B

February 20, 1998

Will:

Today didn't start out too good. I called you around 8:30 AM and the phone has been bad for about a week. You can hear someone else on the phone – you can hear them dialing and talking and there is a lot of air sound – open air. While you were talking I could hear the other party dialing and talking so I told you I couldn't hear you. Well then it started!!! Go get your hearing checked. There's probably something wrong with you.... Will, the stress this time is 100% worse than the first time. Maybe it's because no one is telling us anything and that's because they don't know. I can't take much more. So with you yelling about my hearing I just clammed up. Do you have any idea what's happening here? I have three kids who don't understand why I haven't found a reason for your fever. Why can't we get better doctors, why, why, why? Willie, I'm trying to keep them up and hopeful. I am trying to explain that the doctors do know what they're doing and that the medicine makes you sick and that you will get better. I have your mother calling and crying at me daily. Same questions as the kids and then I have to calm her down and make her believe everything will be okay. Trying to do all this when I honestly don't know what is happening is very stressful. Keeping the house up, paying bills, food shopping, etc. It's getting to me. But – I'll get my hearing checked soon. Yes, I'm upset.

Anyway you had your new shunt put in today. Pat came in with me. You were pretty groggy — morphine, etc. They took you down for your last scan today.

You started to perk up around 3:00 – 3:30 PM. Kathy called to tell us about a scaffolding accident on the 59th Street Bridge. We decided to leave after that — traffic was building. It took us two hours to get home.

I talked to you at night and you seemed pretty good. Oops, they didn't open the line to drip that horrible pre-med stuff. I'll talk to you tomorrow.

Love,

Betty

February 21, 1998

Hi Hon!

Today I didn't get in to see you until later than normal. Will wanted me to stay at his hockey game. He's hoping for another shut out like last week. I got him there at 11:30 and his game was at noon. I stayed for half and the score was 6-1 when I left. The final score was 14-2. They won. I was in your room by 1:00 PM - not bad. You weren't feeling too good. You stayed in bed most of the time. You did get up so I could make your bed. Your nurse, Dina, helped me. She's real nice. I felt like I was on my way out before I knew it. I did finish my book 'The Ghost' today. I left around 4:00 PM. I was supposed to see Kristin tonight - she's been upset lately. But that fell through which was okay with me - I'm tired and don't really feel like going anywhere.

Lana and Alex stopped by just to see how I was holding up. We had chili for dinner (We, being Will and myself).

I talked to you around 9:30 PM - again you didn't sound too great. C'mon Will - it hurts so much to see you like this - I need you.

Love - B

February 22, 1998

Will:

Boy am I tired – I even took a Benedryl hoping to get a good nights sleep. This crazy mind of mine just won't shut off.

Grace and Pat drove in today. Butch was making a pot roast for dinner. I knew you wouldn't want visitors so Pat and Grace walked up to Bloomingdales and to some other store called "Gracious Homes". Something like a Lechter's, but more expensive.

Pat came in to see you around 3:00 PM. Grace had a cough and wasn't sure if it was her asthma acting up or not. She wasn't taking any chances.

You were not good again. When I came in at 12 you were sleeping. I was tired so I fell asleep in the chair for a little bit. You were getting blood. They said you have Cytomegalovirus (CMV). They stopped one of your antibiotics and will slowly stop the rest of your antibiotics and anti-fungal stuff. You didn't eat your breakfast – it was still sitting in your room when I arrived. You did get up and try to eat your lunch. Not too good though. I made your bed and you started with the chills again. I think you had 3 blankets on and the heat was turned up to 78 degrees. I know you hate the chills not only because you said you hate them – but I can see it on your face. Dina was getting ready to hang the blood – and you look like you want to sleep. Besides dying of the heat in your room I had to leave.

Dinner – Kathy, Stephen, Will, Joe and Rocky.

You talked to the kids tonight – Stephen kept nagging me to call you. I didn't get to talk to you for too long – my calling card ran out of time.

I'll talk to you tomorrow.

Love ya lots!

Betty

February 23, 1998

Willie:

Well you looked a little better today. You haven't had a fever in 30 hours or so. That's good. Maybe they found out what's wrong and are treating it with the right stuff. You're still on the amphotericin, but you seem to be handling it better now. The pre-meds really help.

I left when they took you down to Pulmonary – some more tests. I don't know why. You are supposed to have a colonoscopy tomorrow. I went to Jim Johnson's with Kristin. She's a mess. Doug problems. I called you around 10:00 PM. And you were vomiting from the medication they gave you for tomorrow's test/biopsy. You called me back and sounded a little better. You said it was a reaction to the medicine. I feel so bad for you. I'd like to see you have one good day – soon. I'm really tired and my neck is killing me. I used the heating pad for a while, but there was no difference. Hopefully two Advil will take care of it. I'll talk to you in the AM –

Good night love,

B

February 24, 1998

Hi Will –

I talked to you this morning and you didn't sound too great. You had a rough night. They gave you medicine to clean you out for the colonoscopy, but it made you vomit. You also have pain in your shoulder and under your rib cage. They are giving you morphine and Percocet.

When I came in you had oxygen – you said it was because your oxygen level was down. You were very thirsty because you haven't had anything to eat or drink since midnight. You conned me into giving you ice. You look so uncomfortable.

Around 1:30 – 2:00 you went down for a sonogram. They're trying to see what's going on either with your gall bladder, liver or pancreas. You also have a fever of 38.8. While you were having the sonogram Julie came in and said the colonoscopy is going to be tomorrow. You are going to be upset. When you came back I could see the frustration on your face. They should do it in the morning.

I sat down with Dr. Castro today. I asked him how much longer you would be in the hospital and he said 2-3 weeks at least. I can't believe that. I guess I better talk to the kids and let them know what's happening.

I'm really tired so I'm going to bed and will talk to you tomorrow.

Love ya, B

February 25, 1998

Willie:

Today is Ash Wednesday. Today they are going to do the colonoscopy. I'm coming in with Pat. She should be here by 10:30 am. When we got to your room you weren't there. You were still downstairs. When you did come in you were still out of it. You said you wanted an ice cream soda and a black and white. Pat and I walked to 1st and 66th and got you your ice cream soda. You actually drank most of it then your lunch came in and you had some soup.

The rest of the afternoon you slept and snored a lot. Pat and I left around 3:35 PM and were home by 4:45 PM. We had pizza for dinner. I think this is my first Ash Weds since I've known you that I didn't have potato soup and donuts. We'll have it next year.

Stephen freaked on me tonight. Yelling about how he hates everything, hates school, hates teachers...That went on until 11:30 PM. I'm wiped out. Talk to you tomorrow.

Good night,

Betty

February 26, 1998

Willie:

Hi! Again you don't sound good. You seem very tired. I didn't call you until late this morning because I took Kathy to have her stitches removed. I called you about 9:45 and I woke you. You wanted me to call John Mills about Erika's closing. I picked up the papers and bought them in for you to sign.

When I finally got there you were downstairs having an x-ray of your chest. I straightened up your room a bit and drank my coffee. I was watching tv when you came in. You were very tired today. I don't know why though. You didn't really talk to me at all — you slept and I read. I left about 4:10 PM. Tonight was quiet. Rose and Joanne stopped by for about an hour and a half.

I talked to you tonight and you said they want to do a lung biopsy in the morning and drain your lung. What's happening ???

Hon, I'm getting scared!!!!!

Love you,

Betty

February 27, 1998

Will — Right now I'm sitting in your room. I've been sitting here alone since 2:00 PM. You called me this morning and told me that you were having surgery today (lung biopsy). You had me call Al. He said if they see something they should go ahead and be aggressive. His big question was "what about the pain on your side?" You said you wanted me here when you wake up — I'll be here.

I cleaned a little at home — went to Foodtown and made a casserole for the kids, then came to see you. I talked to you at least 1 hour before they took you out of here.

I'll write more later —

It's 11:55 PM. I can't help but to think of how hard it was to leave you. I came down to recovery and stayed about 1 hour. You were really in and out of it today. They had you pretty drugged. Besides the anesthesia (not worn off) they have you on 50 mg of morphine. You have a release button in your hand for the pain. They gave you your pre-meds the Benedryl and Tylenol; they started the drip and half way through they'll give you Demerol.

When I got home (8:45 PM) Grace was here. She wanted to check on the kids and make sure I eat (Pat's instructions). We went to Molly Malone's. We tried to go to Macaroni Grill but there was a line outside at 9:20 so we went up the street. I called you from Molly's and you said you just got up to your room. I called the nurses station when I got home about 10:40 PM. I talked to Cathy. She is your nurse tonight. She said you have a drain in (for a day or two) and a catheter. She said she just came from you and you were sleeping comfortably. I hope that's true. You said you'd call me in the morning – I'll talk to you soon.

Love you Hon–

Betty

February 28, 1998

Will –

Well it's been 3 weeks and we are all missing you here. Get better – PLEASE!!! I know you can't get better on your own, but keep fighting – you have to.

You were really drugged up today. You kept saying funny things. It's weird what goes through your head. You start to wonder if that's the true person coming out. You seemed yourself for five minutes and then you would black out for 2–3 minutes and then you'd say something completely off the wall. You asked me to change the pictures on the wall because you couldn't figure one out. (It was a picture of flowers in a vase on a table). I changed the pictures to a boy drinking from a pond taking sheep to a pasture. You started telling me the sheep were walking under the bridge. There was a dragon in the trees on the right and a monkey in the far right tree. You also told me "I can't believe you won't share" – I just gave you $4800 and you won't share." Then you said I couldn't handle drugs – not like you can – you're doing great!

I came home and did some laundry, cleaned around here and went to Grace's to watch ice skating. I had a salad there. Then I stopped and said hi to Alex and Lana and came home.

I really hate it here any more. I want you home. I need you here. I'll talk to you tomorrow.

Love,

Betty

March 1, 1998

Will –

Today I came in with Pat and Grace. Grace drove, but is still coughing so she didn't come in to see you. She is still not sure if it's allergies or not. She thinks it is because of the forsythia or some other flowers that are starting to bloom.

You are pretty much still out of it from the morphine. You really do say the funniest things.

Before I came, you said you wanted ice cream so we picked that up before we came to see you. You seem to be retaining water now. In fact, you've put weight on. Everyday it's something different. I'm getting scared so you must be too.

You tried to eat lunch, but ended up throwing it up. I hate seeing all of this.

We stayed until 3:30 or so because they are working on the roads and it takes forever to get out. Last night it took me over 2 hrs. to get home.

Butch made a turkey breast for dinner so we ate around 6 PM – cleaned up and everyone left.

The kids want to know when they can come see you. I guess I should bring them in soon. It's almost a month now that you've been here. I never expected any of this.

Hurry home!

Betty

Calls: Sandy, Debi, Al, Mike, Kristin and Nancy.

March 2, 1998

Hi Hon –

I talked to you around 8:45 AM and you said you were sitting in a chair trying to eat your breakfast. You were very short of breath and that was from sitting and answering the phone. You are still on the morphine, but not as heavy a dose. When I got to the hospital I saw your nurse (Fran) who said she gave you a water pill to go to the bathroom because you're gaining weight (water) – not from eating. You threw up your breakfast too. You saw me when I came in – you went to the bathroom and now you are sleeping.

I have to take Magic to the vet at 5:45. She's stinking real bad for some reason. The porch smells so bad everyone holds their breath when they come in. She is drinking her water bowl at least 4 times a day – completely!!. I'll let you know what they say about her.

We went down for another x-ray (chest) about 2:45 PM. I don't understand why they make you go down and then wait forever. We didn't get back upstairs until 4:00 PM. I had five (5) pages from Stephen. Your phone wasn't working. For some reason, it was shut off.

Magic had some blood work done while we were at the vet. I'll get the results Wednesday. Could be liver, kidney or diabetes. I took Stephen to the mall and then helped him clean his closet and drawers.

I talked to you at night. You sounded a little better. I hope you get a good night sleep.

Talk to you in the morning.

Love, B

March 3, 1998

Willie —

Hi — today was a bad day for you. You didn't look too good. While I sat in your room you slept and probably woke up a total of 10 minutes the whole time I was there. You called your mother while I was there. I had myself a pity party. I started thinking how much we've been through since the beginning. First we had the molar pregnancy. Then Stephen being born prematurely 2 ½ months early — the RDS and all we had to go through with him. I remember thinking I wouldn't wish that time on my worst enemy. Then your diagnosis — the medicines, the transplant and now this. I realized my mask was soaking wet. I just sat there looking at you — hurting. I cleaned up my face and put on a new mask. When I got home I cleaned around the house — fed the kids — cleaned out my desk. I talked to you around 10:00 PM and that was my day.

I need you home, hon.

Love ...

March 4, 1998

Will –

This morning seemed to be so hectic. I drove Stephen to school; came home and did some laundry, after my shower I received a a call from Mrs. Flack at HPHS who said Kathy was there with a stomach ache and they needed me to come to the school and follow her home since she had her car. I got Kathy (she's had a bad stomach ache and couldn't stay in school. I then went to Pathmark and came in to see you. You were definitely better today than you were yesterday. You are still on the morphine only because the place where the chest tube was opened again and to keep you comfortable they had you on the morphine for one more day. You haven't showered since Friday – you've been getting sponge baths in bed. Your beard is really heavy now. I think it's heavier than before. After your bath I opened a seltzer flavored water to mix with your coke and it sprayed all over. I got it on you and all over your lunch and floor. I cleaned that up and helped change you. Sorry. You stayed awake a little longer today – I told you about Kristin and Doug. I hope they work their problems out soon.

When I got home, I took Stephen for a haircut – went to the bank, picked Stephen up and took him to the mall to meet Phil and Matt. Then I went to Tops to get cable wire for Stephen's tv. Went to Taco Bell for Will and myself and then to NJ Pet Supply for Magic's breath mints.

I talked to the vet about Magic's blood work. They said her liver enzymes are elevated — it could be caused by bad teeth (which we know she has) but I will talk to Dr. Forester on Monday.

Adrian Connolly called me this evening about Kathy. What the biopsy report showed was a thinning of the skin (happens in young women). It will correct itself over time. He said he would get some cream to me in the next day or so, but it won't clear up overnight. He said it isn't cancerous or lyme disease which it could have been. Thank God.

I talked to you in the evening and you said you were about the same as when I left you. I hope things keep going up hill.

Love, Betty

March 5, 1998

Will –

Hi. Right now I'm sitting at Warnock. I'm having the oil changed on the Jeep. Steve just came in and said they found a torn axle boot and they are going to replace that now. It is covered by the warranty, but it will take another hour or so. I'll write more later.

Continued – March 5, 1998

It is now the evening and I'm finishing today's letter.

After I got home from Warnock (10:15 AM) I had to run to Foodtown to get something for dinner. Pat came a little before 11:00 AM. Pat came in with me today.

You weren't having too good a day, but it wasn't horrible either. You slept most of the time but that was because Julie, your nurse, gave you Ativan for your nausea and it has a sedative in it.

Butch made a flank steak on the grill – it was really good. We had potato puffs and a veggie with it. After Pat and Butch left, Pat Dangler called and I went to Jim Johnson's with them. They wanted to know about you and see how I was doing. (I didn't eat!).

I was home here by 9:00 PM and was going to call you like always around 10:00 PM, but Stephen called at 9:50 PM and needed a ride home from the school play.

I gave you a quick call and asked you to call me back in ½ hour or so. For some reason you said the phone was busy for an hour and finally called me on Will's phone at 11:15 pm. I don't know what was wrong with the phone, but it's been okay since. Talk to you in the morning.

Love,

Betty

March 6, 1998

Will

I hate the end of the week — I'm so tired. I called you this morning and you didn't sound too good. You said you had a lousy night sleep and you kept throwing up. I wish you could eat something — anything!! Grace bought me in today and was going to meet a friend for lunch. We were in the parking garage before 11:30 am. Grace walked up to Bloomingdales and I came up to you. You were sleeping when I came in but woke up about 10 minutes later. You wanted a sip of your apple juice but within minutes your stomach was killing you. You couldn't have any more of your new nausea meds because you had just had it at 10:30 AM. You did get Ativan again today but not until 3:00 pm. Hopefully your stomach will be better.

I talked to you early this evening because I was going to see "Titanic" tonight. I don't know what all the hipe is about — I didn't think it was that great — it's one that will be fine when it comes out on a VCR tape. While I was at the movies I was beeped 4 times total — Ridiculous!!

Talk to you tomorrow,

B

March 7, 1998

Will

Hi! It is now 10:45 PM. It has been one month since you've been home.

Today when I came in your stomach was really bothering you. You moaned for about 20 minutes and then sat up and got sick – bile mostly. I don't think there is anything left in your stomach. Merry gave you something for your stomach and it seemed to work for a while. You tried eating your soup for lunch and you had a little coke. At least they both stayed down. Good sign. You haven't had a fever for 2 days now. Maybe we're on the road to recovery – I hope so.

You also got fresh today, so I know you're getting better you were hot and kicked off your blankets. Then you were cold and tried pulling the cover up but your sheet was all tangled up. I asked if you wanted some help – you said yes and when I tried to help you started to yell because I was under your blanket trying to straighten out the sheet – I walked away and read my book. I understand you are tired of this situation, but it's not that easy for me – really.

I called you this evening and you were trying to have some chicken broth and jello.

I'm bringing Kathy in tomorrow morning and will be back in the afternoon with the Juskins.

See you tomorrow.

Love, – B

March 8, 1998

Will -

Today was the winner. I hope I never get a day like this again.

I called you this morning to tell you Kathy wasn't coming in. She thought Stephen and Will were coming too. She doesn't want to come alone. I thought I would bring them all in one day after school, so I came in alone.

I got to your room early today by 11:30 AM. Within one hour stuff was happening. You were having difficulty breathing, but you of course, don't complain. You said you were okay, but the oxygen level was real low.

Your temperature went up again for some reason. They came in to do blood gases (they hurt - they go into an artery, not a vain). Next someone was there taking an x-ray of your chest.

The x-ray came back with changes no one liked. Fluid in your left lung and maybe a clot. The doctor feels it may be a new pneumonia - a new infection. Another doctor from SCU came in to evaluate, will consult with your doctor and his boss and let us know what's happening.

Merry came in - they're taking you down to the 2nd floor to SCU where they can watch you better. They put a line in so they can do blood gases - at least they won't hurt you anymore. I finally was able to come see you around 7:00 PM. Sherry is your nurse. She's real nice. She came out to me in the waiting room and said, "That guy really loves you. I told him to take off his ring and he did, but he tried putting it on every other finger. I told him I would hold it and he said, No – only Betty." She pinned it to your gown and I took it home. You're sweet, honey.

The Juskins came to see you for about 15 minutes.

Please get better love, you're scaring me.

Love, Betty

March 9, 1998

Willie:

Today was the worst day of my life and probably yours too. I'm not going to write anymore because I know this day will be etched in my memory forever.

Get better, Will — we need you.

Love,

B

March 10, 1998

Will:

I found out yesterday that I cannot handle coming to see you alone anymore. Pat will be coming with me until things get better.

Pat and I got to the hospital around 11:30 am. I am told you are doing better than yesterday. Both Pat and myself cry a lot. To see you this way is so scary. My heart breaks. We changed your radio station, not so "now" music. We changed it to the oldies station. You did hear a couple of Roy Orbison songs. But then our wedding song came on. Yes, I lost it. We didn't turn it off because you seemed to like the radio and if you were subconsciously listening – maybe it gave you a reason to fight. You have a lot of reasons to fight and you better. I can't be alone!

Before we left I went up to the 11th floor to get your last bag. I gave the soda to the nurses. I'm glad we went up because I was able to catch Dr. O'Reilly. He came out and talked to me for a while. Right now no one knows what's happening or where the infection is. I wish they could find it.

I've been talking to your mother every night. I try to explain what's happening as gently as I can. That's tough. She is so upset.

I'm trying to figure out what to do with Kathy, Stephen and Will. They need to come in whether you want them or not. If things get worse, I think they need to see you and say whatever they want. I also think if you see them it will give you another reason to fight. Please don't give up, especially if you see them all around you. It doesn't mean they're here saying good bye. I know if this takes a wrong turn, later on in life they'll say — why didn't you make us go — we were only kids. Sure we didn't want to see him like that, but we needed to..."

We'll see what happens with them. I'll keep you posted.

We're with you, hon — keep fighting.

Love you and need you,

B

March 11, 1998

Hi Will –

Pat and I got to your room before noon. You were definitely more awake I know. Pat and I didn't like to see the frustration in your eyes. You seem to want to say so much. The nurse also wanted to "up" your medication but you were all the way up. She finally had one of the doctors change your sedation medication. I can't remember the name of it, but one of the nurses said it is referred to as "Milk of Amnesia" because of its milky color and you won't remember any of this.

We left the hospital around 3:45 PM. Stephen paged me and said to call Joe Sedges. Joe said he is flying into LaGuardia Airport tonight. He needs to be here for himself – you – me and the kids. I'm not going to stop him, but I don't know what to do with him.

Joe got to the house around 9:00 PM. I wasn't home yet because I went to pick up Kathy's car. They fixed everything. Grace took me up there but she couldn't pick me up until 8 or a little later for some reason. Joe hadn't eaten so we ran over to Jim Johnsons and had a burger and fries. I gave him our room so he has his own bathroom and I'm sleeping with Kathy.

I hope when Joe comes to see you you don't get upset. We'll see you tomorrow –

Love, B

March 12, 1998

Willie:

Pat, Joe and myself came in to see you today. I think you knew who we each are – I hope you know me. Joe said he thought you were better than he anticipated. You were very alert. First you tried talking to us. You then started the charades type of talk. Joe mentioned that you looked good. Your color is good and then you pointed at the tube and everything around you and shook your head as if to say, "yeah, I look real good". Then the nurse and doctor came in and as they were leaving you kept trying to talk. You motioned you wanted a pad and paper to write. Dr. O'Reilly got a pad and pen for you and you started writing – only problem, no one could read it. Dr. O'Reilly told you the meds he was giving you were taking a toll on your penmanship. They want you to rest and save your energy, but you wouldn't stop. Finally you raised your knees and started to write on the sheet like it was a blackboard. Joe told you to write big. You spelled out "ICE. I could have cried – (I did). Just because you were dry from the tube in your throat and it took you 30–45 minutes to get someone to understand you and then we couldn't give you anything because you would choke.

Joe found a sponge swab and wet it then swabbed your mouth, teeth and lips. You seemed happier with that for a little bit.

Next you kept pointing to your wrist. Pat figured you wanted to know what time it was. It was 3:10 PM. You then looked at me with a big question on your face. I then told you it was Thursday — and you couldn't figure out when you came here or why.

We went home today feeling a little more hopeful, yet very upset as to your frustrations. See you later.

Love, Betty

March 13, 1998

Will:

When we got to the hospital you were up to 60% oxygen. This is not good. We need to be going the other way. I'm going to meet with the social worker and with Dr. O'Reilly sometime today. I need to know where things stand and what to do with the kids.

Kathy, Stephen and Will want to see you in a way and then in another way they have some fears, which I understand. I truly feel that fear of the unknown is worse than reality sometimes. I spoke to Pat, the social worker and she said the kids can't be protected forever and they really aren't babies, they are young adults. Joe, Pat and myself sat down with Dr. O'Reilly around 5:00 PM today. He really didn't have too many good things to say. He said you are not getting better daily like he needs you to do. If you reach this medical plateau we're going to be in trouble. You also are not responding to certain new medications. He said if you are going to get better it may be in tiny, tiny little steps, but if things are going to turn, that can happen so quickly.

When I got home, Stephen and Will were there and I paged Kathy. We needed to sit down and let them know what was happening and set up a time to come see you, if they want to.

We explained – I tried and then started crying. Pat and Butch were there, but crying too so Joe S. did the talking. Stephen asked a million questions. Kathy and Will had tears and no questions. They're feelings are mad, scared and angry. We'll all be in tomorrow.

Love, Betty

March 14, 1998

Hi Hon —

Your condition is still stable but there is something in your kidney that is now indicating your kidney is not filtering properly. I think it is something like your creatine level. Something to do with the toxins in your body. Anymore, you are sort of in a clinically induced coma, meaning you can hear but you don't respond to noise or touch too much. You are down to 55% oxygen today — keep fighting Willie. We bought Kathy, Stephen and Will in today. Sherry, your nurse, in fact she admitted you down here last Sunday, came out — talked to the kids and then they came in. Each one was different. Kathy sat in a chair — said Hi Dad — please get better and sat quietly and cried. Stephen kept asking questions and only wants positive answers. Sherry was very good with them. She made sure they understood "Critical" condition but then also gave us all a lot of hope. Stephen did get to a point where he had to leave the room for a few minutes. Joe took him outside. Next Kathy wanted to go so Pat took her out. Will stayed in with me. He was sitting in the chair by your window. I had my back to him, but I noticed he was crying. He needs to get it out. Will is also the only one who got up — held your hand and rubbed your arm and said "Get better, Dad, keep fighting."

Stephen came back in for another 15 minutes or so. Kathy stood outside and just stared and cried. I did explain that whatever feels right for them is fine. There is no right or wrong way to deal with this.

Pat drove the kids home after an hour and a half or so. I think they feel better having seen you. They all said it's not as scary when you know what everything is for.

Ted came in today around 3:00 PM. He was very upset, but he felt better just coming to see you. I spoke to Ted about bringing in your mother and he agreed with the doctors, nurses and social worker — Why put her through it? She can't change anything. Everything around you — ventilator, tubes, monitors, medications, etc. will only scare her.

I know how upset she was when I cut my fingers on Christmas — that doesn't come close to your situation. I can't take anymore emotional stress. I know you won't understand that, but dealing with my feelings and just trying to be there for the kids is wiping me out. I finally figured it out. You want me to look at least your age when my birthday comes around. Guess what? I look your age — ha ha.

Keep fighting my love!

Betty

March 15, 1998

Will:

Today I came in with Joe and he had to go back home by around 1:30. PM. Really his flight isn't until 3:00 but he needs to get back to LaGuardia by 2:00 – 2:15 PM. I told Pat not to come because I wanted some time alone. Not just with you, but myself too. I gave Joe some time alone with you too. That in itself was hard for both Joe and myself. I walked Joe downstairs and he caught a cab and is gone now. He was a great help. We all will miss him.

I came back up to you and sat here writing these letters. Sherry your nurse is great. She talks to you constantly. She tells you how good you look – but tells you to stop scaring us – Fight!! I'm better talking to you through my mind. Who knows – maybe you have mental telepathy and know what I'm saying. I hope so.

Lana and Alex came this afternoon. Alex was very quiet. You can see the pain in his eyes (over the mask). It hurts me to see the pain in all our friends and family's eyes. I can't stand telling people bad news so do me a favor and give me something good to say. We left the hospital about 4:50 pm. Sherry was going to clean you up – turn you to look out the window and make you more comfortable. I also have to get Stephen to CCD class tonight. I'll be in touch with Eileen (your night nurse) before I go to bed and in the AM.

Fight my Love,

Betty

March 16, 1998

Will –

Pat and I arrived at the hospital at about 11:30 AM. I'm glad we got here when we did because Dr. O'Reilly, Alex and Dr. Donnolly just came up too! Your nurse today is Fiona, she's very nice – a real sweetheart, you'd like her.

Dr. O'Reilly just called me out to talk to me. He said that you have reached a plateau and seem to be staying there. You are not responding to the aggressive treatments. What he is doing is he is going to change some meds. So they're not so harsh on your kidney. The toxins are staying in your system, so they won't hurt you by lowering the doses since they stay in your body anyway. He is also going to stop the steroids since there really isn't a change and you've been on them for a while now. He's not going to just "stop" he'll wean you off slowly and see what you do. You better fight like hell!

The kids want to come back in. I'm glad. I'm not sure what day I'll bring them in, but one day this week, I promise. I'm going to go out for a walk now and will write more later.

I'll write tomorrow – I'm too tired now,

Love, B

March 17, 1998

Hi Hon −

Each day is getting harder for both of us. Yes, you are comfortable, but your problems are mounting. The meds are being changed again. You seem to build up resistance to different sedatives and they change them. You are now on a sedative that paralyzes you. I don't really understand why, but Fiona did explain it to me.

When Pat and I came in we were told your lungs are still your main problem. Last night when I called at 10:00 PM your oxygen was up to 65%. Hon, this is not good. When I left in the afternoon it was set at 45% which was okay. They were able to lower it to 60% but they are going back and forth between 60 and 65%. Your blood pressure dropped way down this morning which means your heart is working harder. The drop could be from the change in the meds too.

Will − I know you're fighting your hardest, I just think it's an awful disease you're fighting.

Love you Will −

Betty

March 18, 1998

Will —

Today was the worst trip in ever. Pat left Hackettstown at 9:00 AM and we didn't get to the hospital until 1:50 PM. We sat on the GW Bridge for just under 3 hrs. Every way into the city had problems. There was a jack-knifed tractor trailer that spilled castor oil all over the Cross Bronx Expressway. They closed that and traffic backed up everywhere. We stopped at the 95-NJ Turnpike split. There was an eight mile back up on the Parkway so we didn't try for the tunnel.

When we did finally get to see you it was after 2:00 pm. You haven't had a temperature in 48 hours. That's good. Your kidneys are straightening out. They seem to be putting out enough urine, etc. They came in and did a Doppler of your legs to make sure there are no clots there. They thought that might have been what caused some respiratory problems. Your blood pressure dropped and they gave you certain meds and then you were able to hold you own. I was told it could be from the paralyzing medicine coming out of your body. Your hands and feet are puffy which can be from meds or the infection.

I went home around 5:00 pm and Stephen lost his beeper again. He also lost his keychain. He's so upset with himself. I'm just trying to help him get through this. He says his whole life sucks. I try to tell him that's not true, and just this time sucks. None of our heads are on straight. We can't think of much more than you, which is fine. You are our number one concern right now.

I'm going to sign off. Get better and keep fighting,
Love

Betty

March 19, 1998

Will –

It's really ugly out today. It's only about 36 degrees, rainy and foggy. Grace drove Pat and me in today, just to give us both a break from driving. Grace said to say hello and she said to keep fighting.

Dr. Donnolly and Dr. O'Reilly were in. The CMV is back again. They are treating you with two different treatments. Your kidneys are not a worry anymore and again you don't have a temperature. I think you can do it Will – you have to!!

Dr. O'Reilly said he is still upset with your lungs – you have reached a plateau there. You have to make progress daily – it needs to be just tiny steps – that's okay. Your blood pressure is real low right now. It's 85/40. That's not good Will. You are getting some meds to increase your blood pressure now. They think it's dropping because of the water pill and being used to get rid of fluids. One hell of a big ugly circle. I'm sure we'll find our way out of this mess.

I'll be leaving shortly. I love you, need you and want you Will,

Love,

Betty

March 20, 1998

Will –

For a change we had a very uneventful day coming into the hospital. That was actually nice. We did wait to get into the garage, but not too long – 20 minutes or so.

Your oxygen is up to 70% – that really is not good, Hon. We have to get that down. You've been improving in other areas though. Your fever is back again and your blood pressure is up today. Right now it is 146/55. You seem very cold when I touch you. I asked Diana if I should cover you and she said she doesn't want you covered anymore than you are. She didn't want to turn on the heat lamp above your bed or cover you with more than your sheet. I guess she knows why.

I hope to see Dr. O'Reilly later, just to see what he thinks. I talked to Al yesterday and he said the improvements make him feel a lot better. As long as you make these small improvements, we'll be okay.

The kids call me everyday while I'm here just to calm their minds as to what's happening here. They truly believe you can do anything and you can get over this. God, do I hope they're right! My brother, Bill calls each morning and he's decided to join Stephen's team. He likes the eternal optimist. I'm not saying I'm not optimistic, but I am scared. What will happen to us without you? I'm not even going to go there where things don't go our way. Come back to me Will – please.

Love,

Betty

March 21, 1998

Will

Today when I called in the morning your nurse was busy
with you and they asked me to call back. I called back
about 40 minutes later and she was in with you again
and couldn't talk. I was told you were the same as
last night, no changes. I came in with Pat and we were
there before noon. You weren't the same as last night!
You were up to 100% oxygen. This really is not good,
Will. Al and Joanne came to see you today. Al said
your oxygenation was not good, but your pulse, heart rate
and everything else looked good. The doctors came in
and took me outside and said that it is very grim. They
explained that next to a spinal cord accident, an injured
or sick lung is the worst. I know you are still fighting,
but you are getting tired and I'm so scared.

We went to grab something to eat and we all came back.
Joanne and Al left at about 3:00 pm to head back to
Baltimore. Pat and I stayed until 4:00 pm or so.

Pat dropped me off (asked me if I wanted her to stay,
I said no and she headed home because the weather
calls for snow). I had Will and Dan here and ordered
Chinese food for them. John D. and Pat picked me up
around 7:00 pm to have some pizza. I had 1 slice. We
finished eating and John paid the bill. We were sitting in
Pete's talking when I was paged by the hospital. They
said you weren't doing too good and things were shutting
down. I called Pat and she said she would meet me at

the house. I called Grace, but was never able to reach her. I left a message. John and Pat drove us in and I was with you Will — but only for a few minutes. You waited for me and I thank you for that. I will forever miss you.

I love you!

Betty.

In loving memory of William F. Schaufelberger

October 3, 1947 – March 21, 1997